THE PHENOMENON OF THE SAS IN-THE-CHAIR EXERCISE PROGRAM

It all began with Folke Mossfeldt, the extraordinary Swedish fitness authority . . . and now has become a worldwide phenomenon with thousands of people praising the amazing new fitness program for everyone who sits.

Folke Mossfeldt, fitness adviser to SAS (Scandinavian Airlines), realized that an inflight exercise program would be extremely valuable for everyone forced to spend hours in an airline seat—when freedom of movement is somewhat restricted. He developed a simple but enormously effective series of exercises —and SAS put them into a little booklet for its passengers. It was an immediate and amazingly popular success. SAS could not keep the booklet in print. Thousands and thousands demanded the booklets, including NASA, who thought it would be good for astronauts. Now it's been expanded into book form with new exercises for every conceivable situation. It is, without a doubt, the simplest and best way to keep your body machinery running properly . . . through exercise, when you're forced to sit for hours on end. Enjoy it!

SAS
IN-THE-CHAIR
EXERCISE BOOK

DR. FOLKE MOSSFELDT
AND MARY SUSAN MILLER

BANTAM BOOKS · TORONTO · NEW YORK · LONDON

SAS IN-THE-CHAIR EXERCISE BOOK
A Bantam Book
Bantam edition / March 1979

ISBN 0-553-01163-4

Published simultaneously in the United States and Canada

Bantam Books are published by Bantam Books, Inc. Its trademark, consisting of the words "Bantam Books" and the por-
trayal of a bantam, is Registered in U.S. Patent and Trademark
Office and in other countries. Marca Registrada. Bantam
Books, Inc., 666 Fifth Avenue, New York, New York 10019.

PRINTED IN THE UNITED STATES OF AMERICA

0 9 8 7 6 5 4 3 2 1

Contents

Acknowledgments

The authors give special thanks to Ray Chambers and Gunnar Andersen, whose piloting skills flew them safely through the wild blue yonder of publishing.

I

**Why
This Program
Is
For You**

HOW IT ALL BEGAN

The "No Smoking" sign flashed on. Seat beats clicked to fasten. SAS Flight #912 dipped to land in Stockholm. Between last night's takeoff from Kennedy Airport in New York at 5:05 P.M. New York time and this morning's arrival at Arlanda Airport at 8:45 A.M. Stockholm time, the 375 passengers had sat for eight hours.

Folke Mossfeldt in Seat 24A was impatient for the plane to land. Like the other passengers, he was stiff and weary. His back ached, his feet were swollen, and his head felt groggy. As a frequent traveler, he was used to the exhausting effects of flying, but he was not resigned to them.

Folke Mossfeldt is Sweden's most outstanding physical therapist. He was the expert the royal family called upon some years ago to act as athletic coach for the prince. Twenty years later he saw his former pupil, now King Carl Gustaf, star in the fifty-three-mile, seven-hour Vasloppet Ski Run—a feat only for those in peak physical form. The physical therapist had instilled respect for body training. He felt proud.

It had not been too many years before that the nurses in Stockholm's famed Karolinska Sjukhuset had shaken their heads in alarm, whispering, "Dr. Mossfeldt is crazy." He was treating heart patients in a revolutionary way that he and Professor Torgny Sjostrand had devised. Patients were not to lie immobile in bed for six weeks following a coronary attack, as was customary; they were to get out of bed within five days. Not only get out of bed, they were to climb onto a bicycle and begin exercises.

"We must start building the heart muscle," Folke Mossfeldt explained. The inactivity of lying in bed merely continued weakening it, laying the groundwork for future heart attacks.

Yet here he himself sat on an airplane along with 374 other passengers, inactive for eight hours.

"We are killing ourselves," he thought, "sitting ourselves to death."

He who had added years to the lives of heart patients all over the world was taking years off his own. He who had heard the nurses' mockery turn to worldwide acclaim listened now to self-directed anger.

At this point Folke Mossfeldt made a decision. The plane had landed. He stood up, walked into Arlanda Airport and headed for a phone booth. Two hours later he was sitting again—this time in the offices of Scandinavian Airlines.

Close to a quarter of a million people fly from New York to Stockholm on SAS every year. Dr. Mossfeldt pointed out that each of those passengers suffers boredom, fatigue and physical harm directly due to the long flight.

SAS executives agreed but countered with the fact that the millions of passengers who fly on all airlines to other parts of the world suffer equally.

"SAS can be different." He spoke of a solution. He envisioned a program aimed at stimulating the flow of blood from the heart to all muscles of the body, even those at the extremities. This would entail large-muscle exercises to put the heart to work and small-muscle exercises to stimulate localized areas such as feet, hands and neck.

The executives listened as Dr. Mossfeldt outlined a program, explaining how exercises could be done while sitting in the airplane seat—even with the seat belt fastened. They asked questions.

"Do you think people would really do the exercises?"

"They wouldn't dare *not* do them if you explain the reason."

The executives nodded in approval. Then came the clincher.

"Would these exercises really do any good?"

Folke jumped to his feet. "That I promise."

And so the program was born: Exercises in the Chair. Folke Mossfeldt designed them. Kerstin Olsson and Lars-Arne Hult illustrated them. And passengers from all over the world went crazy over them.

Then nonpassengers from all over the world went crazy over them.

The original print order of 250,000 brochures vanished in the air like a jet stream. A second print order followed suit. Response to the brochure, now in its third printing, still has SAS executives stunned.

"We're not in the publishing business," they gasp.

The idea has been copied, borrowed and rented. It has been envied, reported and spread by word of mouth. Tens of thousands of brochures have been mailed to doctors, nurses, convalescents, businessmen, housewives and students. Corporations such as Ford and Westinghouse have ordered additional tens of thousands. Even the U.S. government has gotten into the act. NASA asked for 100 brochures to relieve the space-sitting tedium of astronauts in training. And way up in Iceland, 200 soldiers manning the Defense Early Warning Line are exercising in the chair as they keep watch on the skies.

What began as a way to keep feet from swelling on an airplane has become a national craze—with good reason. Americans have come to realize that even if they never fly, they sit for even longer periods of time and with much greater frequency in their everyday lives.

PEOPLE DO A LOT OF SITTING

The city dweller spends about ten hours a week commuting to work on subways and buses and in automobiles.

The county dweller, depending solely on a car for transportation, sits almost fifteen hours a week behind the wheel.

The suburbanite spends up to twenty hours a week getting from a bedroom community to the office.

Business executives sit at the desk or conference table eight hours a day.

The secretary's sitting hours are the same—at steno pad, phone and typewriter.

Students sit in class and at homework six hours a day.

Teachers sit the same six hours while preparing lessons and correcting papers.

Moviegoers average four hours in plush seats every week.

Women sit about an hour and a half a week in beauty parlors; men, somewhat less—despite unisex.

Husbands sit and read the paper; wives sit and read, knit and write letters; together they sit and play records, go to church and visit friends—a minimum of ten hours a week.

Everybody sits and eats—a particularly lethal combination of activities—twenty hours a week, not counting snacking time.

When five o'clock rolls around, America becomes a virtual game of musical chairs. People rush from their professional sitting spots to other seats—at bars, at kitchen tables and on assorted means of transportation.

This long list of sedentary hours does not even include the greatest put-down of all: television. Americans sit in front of their TV sets an average of forty hours a week—more on weekends watching football, baseball, basketball and hockey. On Thanksgiving and New Year's Day it is possible, because of the country's time zone differences, to sit for twelve hours atrophied before the dim blue light and the cheers of fans in the stadium.

SAS Exercises in the Chair speaks, you might say, to America's bottom line.

It was this bottom line that Dr. Mossfeldt tallied on the plane when he realized that people were sitting themselves to death.

THE MACHINE BUILT TO LAST 150 YEARS— YOUR BODY

Modern lives depend on machines, on an assortment as varied in size as a jumbo jet and a pocket calculator; as varied in use as a microwave oven, a typewriter and a transistor radio. We buy them, we follow directions for their care, we have them repaired when parts wear out, and we turn them in for new models, complaining lightly that "they don't make things the way they used to."

Yet the machine on which we depend most heavily —our body—receives little thought or attention. It is built to outlast all other machines. It has not become obsolete in close to a million years. Yet we toss it few compliments, and we give it little care.

SAS Exercises in the Chair helps you do both. With this book you will come to respect the wondrous machine that is your body. You will learn how, in only a few minutes a day, you can keep it in top condition—smooth and long-running.

Our body does for us what can be done only by many other machines combined. It moves us, lifts and reaches and grasps. It responds and communicates. It solves problems. It creates and protects. It recharges itself. It even reproduces.

Most wondrous of all, the body adjusts itself to

meet our changing needs. When the temperature is 40 below or 120 above, the body manages to stay at 98.6. When there is infection, it sends white blood cells to heal. When the surface is cold, it shudders, drawing red blood cells to warm. When it is hot, it perspires for cooling evaporation. It blinks to keep dirt out of the eyes. It regurgitates food alien to the stomach. It eliminates excess fluid and waste matter. It faints to avoid shock. It grows back the nails and hair and outer skin lost in the bustle of living. Our body takes a lot of abuse and only occasionally falls apart in inconvenient places such as the tennis court or jogging path. Most of the time it transports us dutifully to the chairs and beds in which, as we have already seen, we spend too much of our time.

For fuel the body requires a balanced diet but continues to operate on the unbalanced one we feed it. It keeps going despite the martinis and cigarette smoke we pour into it and battles its way bravely through the soot-thick, chemical-heavy air it is forced to breathe.

The young take the body for granted. The middle-aged pretend it is not there. Only the old, as parts disintegrate and pains set in, realize its lost efficiency. They marvel at what was. They philosophize on the all too short seven ages of man. And soon they die. Too soon. Needlessly soon.

Death is a kind of suicide, self-inflicted ahead of time. For this machine, this body of ours, is built to last 150 years—with parts strong and operative. What it needs is care, the kind of care we give our other machines.

Care includes two basic ingredients. One is fuel; the other is proper use. Our body's fuel is the food, liquid and gases we take in. Our body's proper use is the activity to which we subject it. This book concerns the latter. Our purpose is to show that even in the sedentary lives we lead, we can give our body much of the activity it requires for peak efficiency and long life.

WHAT MAKES
THE BODY RUN?

Let us look at this machine on which our life depends. Let us put it in the garage, as it were, remove the hood, keep the motor running, and watch it operate.

It is a network of systems, interrelated, yet each controlled by its own parts or organs.

The digestive system handles fuel, which, like gas station attendants, we pump through the mouth. The stomach selects what the body can use, sending off the rest as waste through the kidneys and colon.

Thousands of muscle fibers throughout the body move us. However, with no mind of their own, they rely on our brain to give them directions. The nervous system with its gossamer threads takes the directions. It carries the message from brain to muscle, directing itself to the particular muscle that is being called upon to perform. The muscle obeys and moves us in the direction our brain wills.

The respiratory system brings in the ingredient most crucial to life: oxygen. Without this, we cannot live more than a few minutes. With every breath, the lungs—balloonlike—fill up with inhaled air. They separate oxygen for use in the body and send back through exhalation other components of air that we cannot use.

The reproductive system, which for reasons known only to Adam and Eve as they reached for fig leaves, has long been considered off limits. Highly efficient, it is the one system that is used far less often for its assigned duty than for pure pleasure—which gives the body a distinct advantage over other machines.

Each of these four systems, busy in its twenty-four-hour-a-day specialized job, depends on a fifth system: the circulation. This fifth system is what *SAS Exercises in the Chair* is all about. For the circulation has the job of feeding the rest of the body, of keeping it alive. To do this, it needs the daily activity this book outlines.

The circulatory system works like a trucking operation, delivering on demand what over sixty trillion cells order and returning what they do not want. For instance, it drops off calcium to the bones, salt to the muscles, iodine to the thyroid, vitamin A to the eye, vitamin K to the liver, etc. It returns nitrogen, uric acid, and materials in excess such as sugar and salts. Most important, the circulation works in conjunction with the respiratory system to deliver oxygen. Just as we cannot live beyond a few minutes without breathing to bring air into the lungs, so we cannot live beyond a few minutes without circulating oxygen throughout the body.

Seventy-five thousand miles of blood vessels operate within a person's body. That is more miles than SAS covers in all its flights combined—or that any global airline flies.

The delivery begins in large arteries carrying red blood, rich in supplies. It extends through the network of branching arteries, getting smaller and smaller and smaller until it reaches the thinnest capillaries at the body's extremities. Here, by an exchange of fluids by osmosis, the delivery is received by cells, and the waste is returned.

The process is then reversed. The bluish, nonnutritious blood returns from cells into capillaries, through small veins converging to larger ones. It finally reaches the heart or the lungs for recharging or dies and is discharged along the way. The entire circuit takes a mere fifteen seconds.

YOUR HEART—
THE IRREPLACEABLE MOTOR

The motor that keeps this cycle going is the heart. Nothing that has been said of this organ—be it in love songs, lace valentines or anatomy books—can do it justice. The heart is the closest nature comes to perfection. Inventions that win Nobel Prizes pale in comparison. Spaceships are as simple as toy gliders beside it. Tomorrow's robots are more comprehensible and less awesome than the heart that beats in each of us.

Lodged in the chest, the heart is a muscle—triangular in shape, with the lower, narrower end pointing toward the left. It is about six inches long, four inches at the widest, and weighs about twelve ounces. During the day it beats an average of sixty to eighty times a minute, as indicated by one's pulse. During the restorative hours of sleep, it beats about fifty to sixty times a minute.

Like all muscles, it depends upon oxygen from the blood to sustain it. Unlike other muscles, however, which rely on outside sources to feed them, the heart feeds itself. Like a garden fountain that recycles water, the heart recycles blood. It allows for no waste.

The heart performs its work through four sections into which it is divided: two receiving chambers—the atria—on top, and two pumping chambers—the ventricles—on the bottom. The left atrium receives nutritious blood from the lungs and passes it through a valve into the left ventricle, which in turn pumps it through the body. After body cells take out the ingredients they want, the blood—now nonnutritious —returns to the right atrium. From there it passes through a valve to the right ventricle and is pumped into the lungs. It has made a complete circuit of the body.

In the lungs the blood is recharged with oxygen, to return to the left atrium, where the whole circuit began—and begins again and again and again. It begins a hundred thousand times a day, pumping over ten thousand quarts of blood.

Filling this job description, the heart is by far the strongest muscle in the body. In the least of us, it does more than Mohammed Ali's jabbing biceps, than Arnold Schwarzenegger's weight-lifting chest muscles, than Rudolph Nureyev's leaping gluteals, than O. J. Simpson's touchdown-running thighs.

Great as the heart is, however, it has one flaw. Unlike many muscles, it can neither repair nor replace itself. Once damaged, it remains damaged. Once a part of it is destroyed, that part never again functions as before. Scar tissue forms, allowing the rest of the heart to work, but never as fully as before —more like a six-cylinder car running on five cylinders.

Young people give little thought to heart damage, despite the fact that it begins to set in as early as the mid-twenties. The middle-aged, however, are shocked into awareness. Jim Sommers, a neighbor, forty-eight years old, drops dead on the tennis court. Bill Evans, a friend, fifty-two, collapses while shoveling snow. Art Weber, a business associate, fifty-seven, dies behind his desk.

The life-span has lengthened by fifteen years since the 1920s. Infectious diseases have been virtually wiped out. Infant mortality has been cut dramatically. Diabetes is under control. New drugs handle pneumonia, syphilis, and tuberculosis. Yet heart diseases are as fatal as ever. In civilized countries around the world, heart disease is the number one killer. Finland and the United States lead the way; Sweden, an activity-oriented country, is notably near the bottom of the list.

WHAT SITTING DOES TO YOUR BODY

Let us, while this body is in the garage with the hood up, take a look and decide for ourselves.

What happens to the body when it sits?

1. The heart slows down on the job—less work is demanded, less work is done. Thus:

• The heart muscle becomes weaker, less able to pump strongly when the body reactivates itself.

• Blood circulates more slowly through the vessels, enabling deposits to form in arteries.

• High blood pressure may ensue.

• The groundwork is laid for coronary thrombosis.

2. Muscle pumps throughout the body, whose job it is to force blood back up to the heart, relax and weaken. Thus:

• Gravity takes over, and legs, hands, and feet swell with collected blood.

• Varicose veins may form from pools of blood that settle instead of flow.

3. The supply of oxygen required to feed the body's muscle cells is curtailed by the inadequate flow of blood, the oxygen-carrier. Thus:

• Muscles stiffen and ache.

• Muscles atrophy, eventually becoming unusable.

4. With the full body's weight resting on the base of the spine, pressure is exerted incorrectly. (Man is a standing animal.) Thus:

- Back and stomach muscles sag, causing all-too-common lower back pains and poor digestion.
- With too little blood circulating to the spinal muscles, they tend to spasm.

5. During a long sitting period, shoulders and neck remain inactive. Thus:

- The top four vertebrae grow stiff from inactivity. A typical "dowager's hump" may form.
- Muscles tense, causing stiff neck and headache (most noticeable when you drive a car for a long period of time).
- The liquid that lubricates the body's joints is produced only through movement. This liquid prevents the discs of the vertebrae from rubbing against each other. Motionless sitting causes the vertebrae to dry and spinal problems to follow.
- Both the dryness and the tenseness may trigger arthritis.

6. The brain, fed by blood as the rest of the body is, receives an insufficient supply during inactivity. Thus:

- It becomes logy.
- When you suddenly stand after long sitting, you become dizzy as gravity pulls blood away from the brain and your circulation is too inactive to resist the pull.

7. Since the condition of body reflects that of mind, and the condition of mind reflects that of body, long sitting shrouds both in low-key depression. Emotional and physical vigor dissipate.

ARE YOU SITTING
YOURSELF TO DEATH?

However uncomfortable and enervating these effects of oversitting may be, it is worth taking a closer look at the actual disasters contained within them.

What happens inside our sedentary bodies is what happens inside the water pipes in our home. When water is running in the pipes, we have no problems: the kitchen sink fills, the shower sprays, the toilet flushes. In the warmth of summer we do not even think about it. In winter, however, as the temperature falls below thirty-two degrees, we hope for good radiators and thick insulation. Without them the pipes will freeze solid—unless we keep water gushing through them full force twenty-four hours a day. On this principle Niagara Falls does not freeze over —but Lake Ontario does. Flowing water.

So it is with our blood vessels. Although genetics, diet, stress, and smoking contribute to hardening of the arteries, each of us can overcome the deleterious effects through exercise. If we keep blood rushing through our arteries—like Niagara Falls—we have a far better chance of keeping them open. But when the flow becomes slow motion—like Lake Ontario— deposits called plaque form on the walls. These thicken the walls, lessen the artery's opening, and cut down on the amount of blood delivered to the tissues. Eventually the artery closes completely, cutting off its blood supply to the dependent tissue, which then dies of starvation.

Arteries may also be blocked by clots, which are another damaging result of inactivity. A continual rush of blood wears away clots as they begin to form —as rushing water.wears away ice. In the slow-moving bloodstream, however, clots may build up and eventually obstruct the flow of blood completely.

Unlike water pipes, arteries can be trained to handle their blockage during periods of activity. They put into operation new arteries, which carry blood around the blocked one. In effect, blood is enabled to continue on its route by a detour around the damaged part of the artery and back into it where it is still open. This process is awesome evidence of the body machine's adaptability. But—and this is a large *but*—this compensatory artery-building can take place only in an active body, not in one that sits.

When the blood supply to muscles other than the heart is cut off, the result is the soreness and stiffness associated with old age—morning aches, bent posture, lost energy. It may, however, be more serious.

Imagine a gallon of water pumped at the same rate through two pipes—one an inch in diameter, the other a quarter of an inch. In the larger one, the flow of water will be easy. In the smaller one, it will be forced through under great pressure.

The smaller pipe is your plaque-filled artery, through which it is more difficult for blood to flow. The heart, therefore, must pump harder. The result is an overworked heart muscle and often an artery bursting under pressure for which it was not built.

When the blood supply to a part of the brain is cut off—by either a clot or deposits of plaque—that part of the brain receives no oxygen. The result is what we call a stroke: The affected area of the brain becomes inoperative. Nerve messages assigned to that area cannot be carried, and paralysis occurs.

When the blood supply to the heart is cut off, results are even more lethal:

1. Thickened arteries lessening the flow to the heart cause angina—the heart's painful screaming for oxygen.

2. When one muscle in the heart becomes weaker than the others, the balance of blood intake and output is thrown off. The lungs receive more blood than they can send back into the heart, and in effect they drown. This balance is so delicate that even one drop of blood more per pump will congest the lungs in a few hours.

3. Total blockage of one of the heart's arteries causes coronary thrombosis. This is death of a muscle and causes irreparable damage to the heart. If only a small section of the muscle is involved, scar tissue will form, and the heart will continue to function. If, however, a large area of the heart has deadened, the heart cannot perform its job. With the circulatory system malfunctioning, the interrelated body systems fall instantly apart. The result is death.

Have we then answered the question: "What happens when we sit?" In answering that one, have we not also answered our other question: "Are we sitting ourselves to death?"

We have seen the damage that endless hours of sitting can do—from the minor backache to the major heart attack. It follows, therefore, that exercise can prevent many of the circulatory problems we see resulting in obituaries we read.

"Then how come Jim Sommers dropped dead on the tennis court?"

Because Jim Sommers did not exercise. He went on a weekend binge. No exercise at all is safer than sporadic exercise. With no exercise, a person's circulatory system adapts itself to a slow crawl. The heart pumps lethargically; the blood flows weakly. The person sits back, dying slowly but surely as arteries thicken and close.

To take the body that sits all week, however, and throw it headlong into a tennis match on Saturday means dying just as surely but less slowly. The slow-motion circulatory system is suddenly called upon to provide fast-motion blood to muscles in action. Ill equipped, it shoots a clot to the heart or bursts a vessel or overtaxes a scarred ventricle.

Only a person who favors his body with an exercise program can handle the spurt of activity. A program involves two factors: (1) activity that is regular —not the usual five-minute morning routine or Saturday tennis match, but exercise built into the entire day; (2) activity that involves both large and small muscles in all parts of the body in a medically sound way.

While the ideal program might involve a mile of jogging every other hour, we have seen earlier that the daily routine of our life does not allow for this. We have work to do—most of it, sitting-down work. However, if we do not put these sedentary hours to active use, we shall, like the passengers on the airplane, sit ourselves to death.

II

How to
Use
This Book

FOLLOW THE PROGRAM

All Day
Any Place
Any Time

SAS Exercises in the Chair lets you adapt movement to your personal sedentary routine every day, all day long, whether at home, at work, or on the town. It lets you live better while sitting at the kitchen table, at your desk, or at a movie. Although the illustrations are set in an airplane, in a car, in front of the television set, on a train, at the office, and in a waiting room, you can do them wherever you happen to be —any place, any time.

The following pages offer a wide variety of exercises. They are presented in seven different units— programs A through G. Programs A and B are full exercise programs, involving all areas of the body. Programs C through G, equally important, offer alternative exercises that will prevent your getting bored and will, at the same time, stimulate circulation and exercise muscles.

For best results do the exercises as follows:

1. Select whichever exercise unit you want to do (A through G). Vary them from time to time, depending on the body area you want to work on.

2. Always begin with a warm-up, which activates the body's large muscles (see exercises A1, B1, C1, D1, E1, F1, G1). This gets blood flowing to all muscles of the body and at the same time, limbers them so they will not tear during exercise.

3. Next, speed up your circulation (see exercises A8, B2, B7). This provides nourishment to the muscles you will be exercising. It also strengthens muscle pumps so they can force blood from the extremities back to the heart.

4. Now work on your specific muscles:

Back and stomach
(see exercises A5, C2, D2, E2, F2, G2).

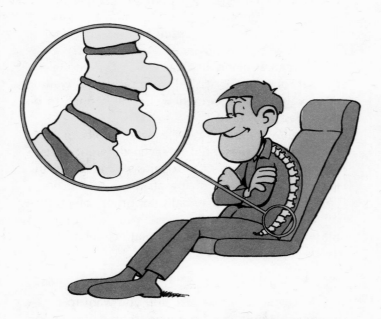

A. With your spine erect, vertebrae discs remain lubricated and properly positioned.

Here you strengthen muscles that hold the back and spine erect, thus enabling yourself to develop good sitting habits. As a result, you avoid the lower back problems from which 80 percent of Americans suffer at some time. With your spine held erect and the blood flowing, vertebrae discs remain lubricated and properly positioned. Thus you avoid irritations that cause joint diseases. At the same time, you build muscles to hold the stomach firm—a corset of muscles, in effect. This, through pressure on the stomach and intestines, aids digestion and bowel regularity.

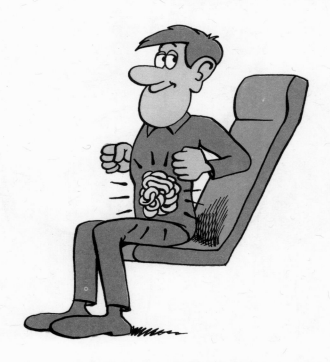

B.   An erect spine also builds muscles
to hold the stomach firm.

Shoulders
(see exercises A3, B3, B6, C3, D3, E3, F3, G3).

Proper shoulder movement stimulates the fluid that keeps joints lubricated. Bursitis and arthritis are far less likely to be triggered. In addition, shoulder exercise activates upper back muscles, preventing stiffness and soreness commonly resulting from over-sitting.

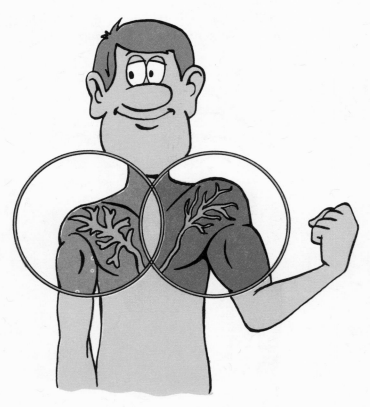

C. Proper shoulder movement stimulates the fluid that keeps joints lubricated.

Neck (see exercises A4, B4, C4, D4, E4, F4, G4).

People usually move their neck so slightly and so incorrectly as to put only the first vertebra to work. These neck exercises help you move—and move correctly—not only the first but the second, third, and fourth vertebrae as well. This relieves tension, which causes the world's most common complaint: headache. It also keeps the upper spine flexible.

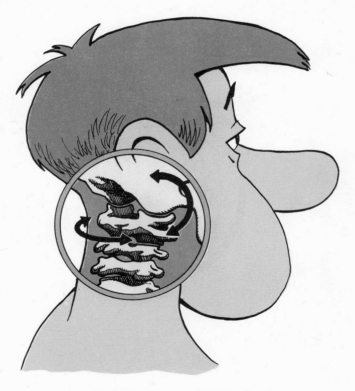

D. Neck exercises can relieve the world's most common complaint: the headache.

Feet (see exercise A7).

This lubricates ankle joints to prevent stiffness and pain. It also aids in preventing swelling of the legs and feet.

Legs (see exercises A2, B5).

This keeps leg muscles from stiffening during inactivity. It also prevents swollen legs by speeding up blood flow to resist the pull of gravity. Blood does not settle in the legs.

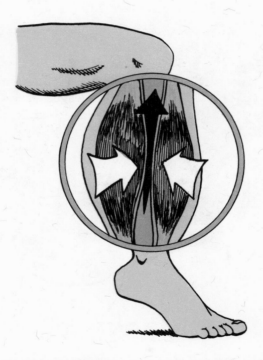

E. Exercises keep the legs from stiffening and swelling.

Hands (see exercise A6).

This lubricates wrists and finger joints, which are the prime targets for arthritis. It also helps prevent swelling of the fingers by forcing the blood upstream.

If at first you are shy about doing the exercises in public, you may seek a quiet corner where you can do them unobtrusively or turn your back to the crowd or find an exercise-mate to share them with you. However, as you discover the new, physically fit you that emerges, you will gain confidence.

"Won't you join me?" you may ask as you jog in place on the subway.

"Have you tried this one?" you may suggest to the mother in the park.

Many Swedish companies have a staff member who goes from office to office organizing exercises for employees. Perhaps your colleague at the conference table or your secretary rising from her typewriter, maybe the mail boy or the president of the conglomerate will surprise you tomorrow by saying, "Let's take an exercise break."

As you look up from your chair, don't just sit there. Join him.

HOW YOUR BODY RESPONDS

In the process of moving your body muscles as the program guides you, you are exercising your number one muscle: the heart. You are making it strong. You are keeping your circulation busy. You are building new arteries as backups for those arteries that may through age or disease be put out of commission.

You have not even moved from your chair. You are still talking on the telephone, watching the baby, dictating a letter, riding in a car, taking notes in class. However, you have refused to waste your time and waste your body. You have learned to sit and to live at the same time.

So now

- your blood keeps flowing.
- your heart keeps pumping.
- your muscles keep working.

There is far less chance of

- plaque forming.
- clots building up.
- stroke.
- coronary thrombosis.
- angina.
- high blood pressure.
- spinal problems.

- arthritis.
- headache.

You notice

- easier breathing.
- less stiffness and aching.
- more energy.
- greater sense of well-being.

You have

- slowed down the aging process.
- toned up your body.
- made weekend activity safer.
- in short, made life better.

The Old Testament prophet Isaiah described the enemy as "those who sit still."

In reading *Exercises in the Chair* you have seen the enemy—and it is you.

In doing Exercises in the Chair you have overcome the enemy. You are the victor.

EXERCISE PROGRAM
A

1. Jogging on the spot.

A warming-up exercise.

It makes sense to warm up properly before strenuous exercise. Use simple, rhythmic movements, engaging as many muscle groups as possible. "Jog on the spot" by raising your heels alternately as high as possible. At the same time raise your arms in a bent position, and rock rhythmically forward and back as when walking. Continue one to three minutes.

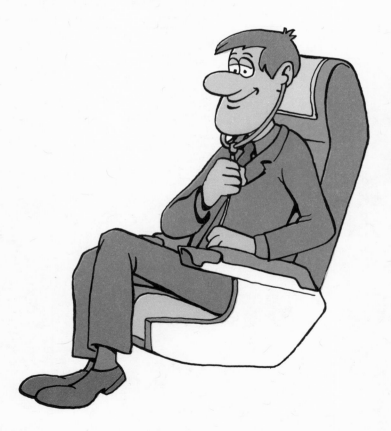

2. Raising on the toes.

Improves blood circulation to the legs.

Sit with elbows on knees, bending forward with your whole weight pressed down on the knees. Lift up on toes with the heels as high as possible. Drop heels and lift toes. Repeat the whole exercise thirty times.

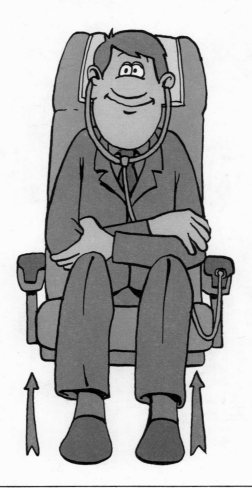

3. Shoulder rolling.

Stimulates the joints, relaxes shoulder muscles.

Joints thrive on regular motion. Smooth, rhythmic movements "lubricate" the inner joint. Move the shoulders gently and rhythmically, at intervals, describing large circles in both forward and backward directions.

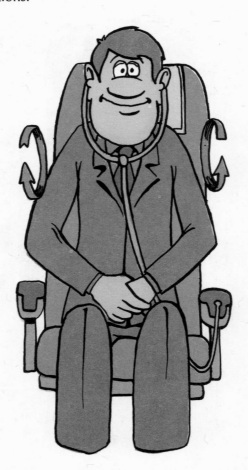

4. Head turning and nodding.

Stimulates joint capsules and cartilage in upper spinal column.

It is important to regularly activate the joints to the full extent of movement. Occasionally do the following: Turn the head the fullest extent to the right. Nod a few times. Do the same toward the left. Repeat the entire exercise six times.

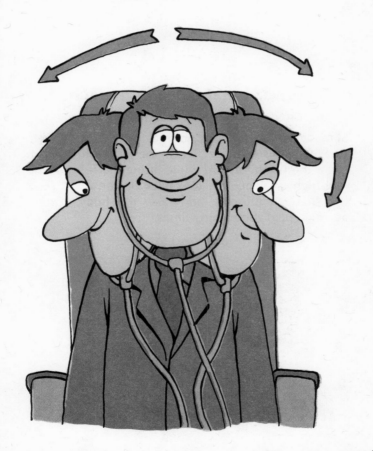

5. Forward bends with stomach in.

Stimulates bowels and blood circulation.

Stimulate blood circulation and improve the digestion with this exercise: Draw the stomach fully in.
Drop the trunk forward while lifting the front of the
feet high up. Place the toes back on the floor, relax
the stomach muscles, and raise the body upright
again. Repeat about thirty times.

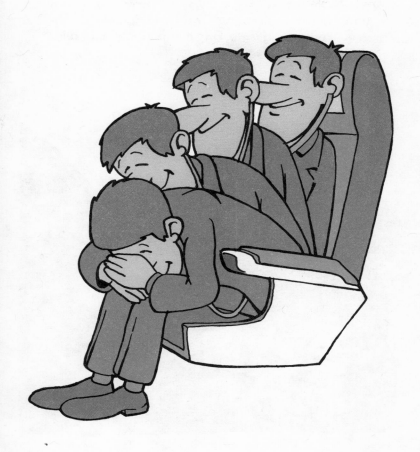

6. Hand turning.

Stimulates the wrists.

The cartilages and joint capsules in the wrists also need stimulation. A good way to achieve this is to turn the hands all the way over and spread the fingers. Return hands to original position and relax them. Repeat fifteen times.

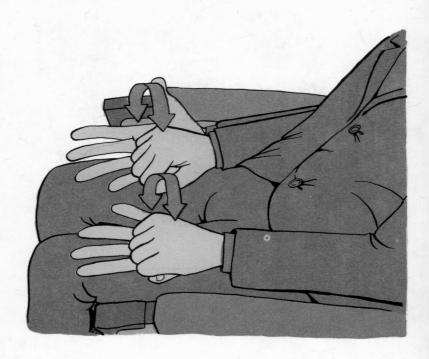

7. Foot rolling.

Stimulates the ankles.

Exercising the ankle joints now and again by rolling the feet in large circles to the full extent of their movement is a valuable form of stimulation. Repeat fifteen times in each direction.

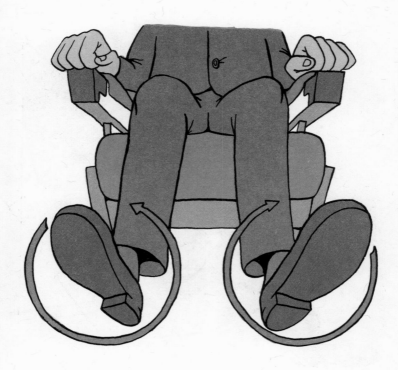

8. Knees up against the elbows.

Speeds up blood circulation.

Now and then, preferably at regular intervals, one should increase the blood circulation by setting to work large groups of muscles. This is one way: Drive the left and right knees alternately up toward the opposite elbow. Repeat fifteen times in each direction.

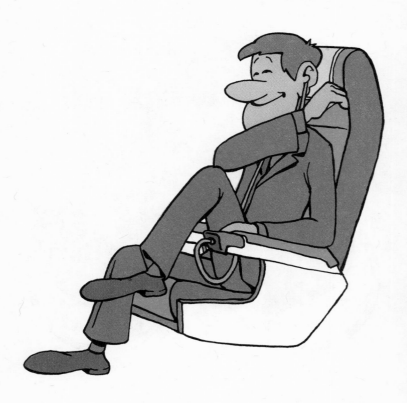

EXERCISE PROGRAM
B

1. Rowing while seated.

A warming-up exercise.

This warm-up session takes the form of an imaginary "rowing" action. Stretch the arms forward while bending the upper body forward for a rowing "stroke." Lift the forward part of the feet right up, then press down the toes, draw in the arms, and at the same time move the body backward, completing the "stroke." Repeat the exercise for one to three minutes.

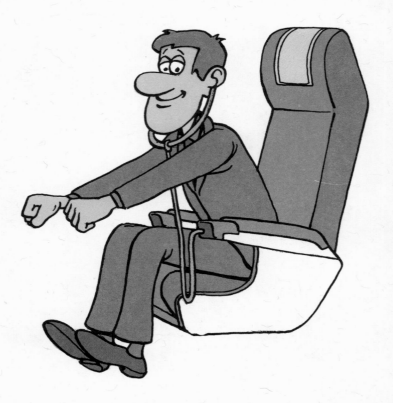

2. Alternate knee raising.

Speeds blood circulation.

In this exercise we speed up the blood circulation and flow by lifting the left, right, and finally both legs in succession. Grasp the hands together and "pull." Repeat the exercise ten times each for left, right, and both legs.

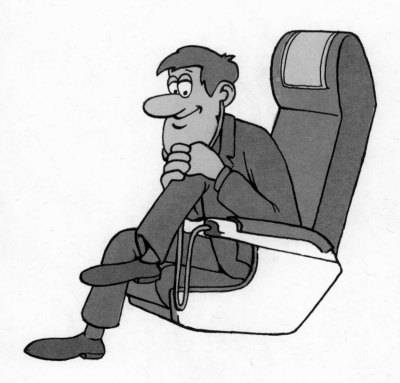

3. Apple picking.

Stimulates the shoulders.

The shoulder muscles and joints are stimulated by alternately and rhythmically stretching up the arms as if picking fruit from a tree. This exercise is alternated with a rhythmic movement of the shoulders forward and back, holding them in a dropped, relaxed position. Repeat the exercise ten times with each arm and the shoulders.

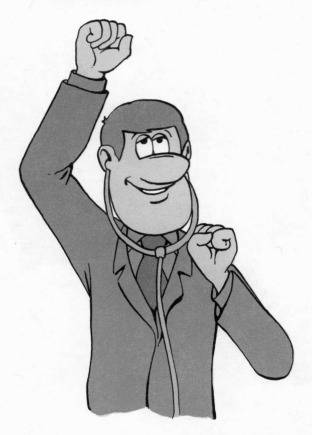

4. Alternate head turning.

Stimulates joint capsules and cartilage in upper spinal column.

Bend the head forward (chin against the throat). Keep the chin against the throat and "bend" the head backward. Turn the head as far as you can to the right and nod three times. Return the head to the front. Do the same toward the left. Repeat the whole exercise ten times.

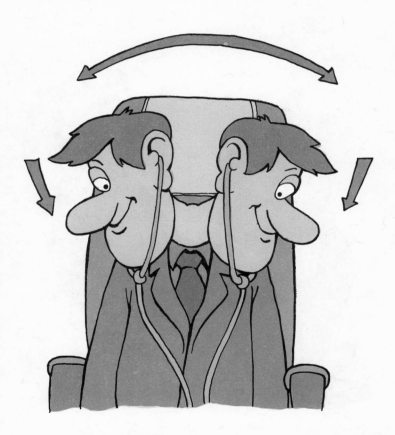

5. Rising and sitting.

Improves flow of blood to legs and blood circulation.

Speed up circulation and stimulate the passage of blood to the legs with this exercise: Gently rise upward or attempt to rise, with or without the help of the hands. Sit down again and lift the toes. Repeat the exercise thirty times.

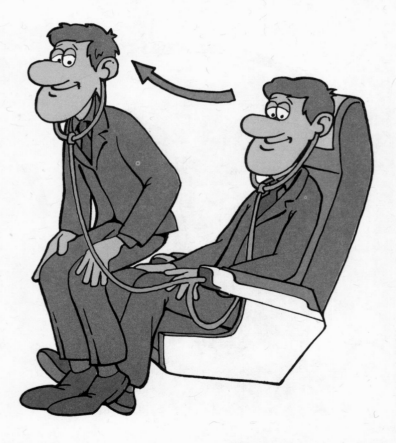

6. Double arm-swings.

Stimulates the shoulders.

To stimulate the muscles and joints of the shoulders and elbows: Sit with the hands clasped. Swing the arms gently, rhythmically upward and backward, stretching them while turning the palms upward. Bring the arms down again and relax. Repeat the exercise ten to twenty times.

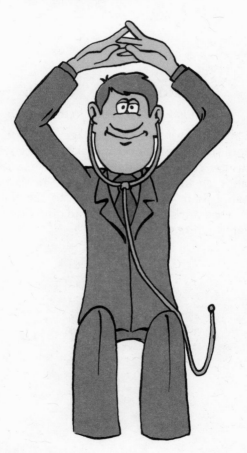

7. Slalom while seated.

Stimulates the blood circulation.

Slalom-skiing improves the passage of blood to the legs and stimulates blood circulation. Sit with the heels as far out to the right as possible, with both the hands on the same side. Lift the heels right up and swing them all the way over to the left while swinging the arms over in the same direction. Repeat the exercise thirty times.

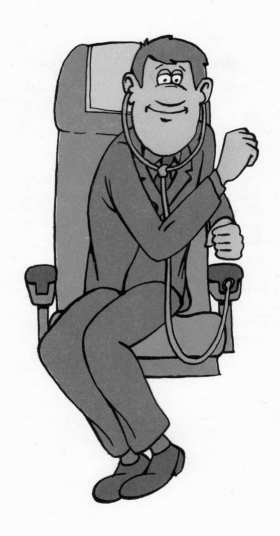

8. Relaxation. Muscle control.

We often tense various muscles unnecessarily for short or long periods, sometimes without realising it. Training for muscle control and relaxation technique helps counteract this and is beneficial in other ways. Try this exercise: Sit fully relaxed. Breathe evenly and gently using so-called diaphragm breathing. This involves filling the stomach when breathing in, which is an active motion. On breathing out, which is a passive motion, the air is slowly released and the body sinks into complete relaxation.

In order to become aware of the difference between tensed and relaxed muscles, and to avoid unnecessary tensing, as mentioned above, practice alternately tensing and relaxing various muscle groups. Repeat the exercise until you feel heavy, pleasantly relaxed.

EXERCISE PROGRAM

C

In the Car

1. With your right foot on the gas pedal, press your left heel against the floor as hard as possible. Pull the toes toward you, tensing the ankle. Now move your foot under your body, putting weight on the toes and pushing the ankle forward. Repeat thirty times. (If not driving, do the exercise with both feet —although doing it with only one foot helps circulation in the other.)

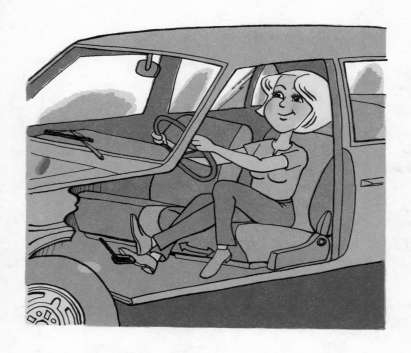

2. Sit relaxed. Raise the back through a concentrated pulling together and tensing of the lower back muscles. Shoulders should remain dropped. Keep the muscles tensed for seven seconds. Relax for seven seconds. Repeat the exercise eight times.

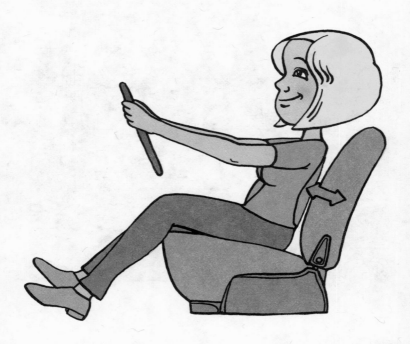

3. Sit with shoulders dropped. Pull the left shoulder as far up as you can. Tense. Drop. Relax. Do the same with the right shoulder. Repeat the whole exercise twice with both shoulders together. Repeat exercises for left, right, and both shoulders eight times.

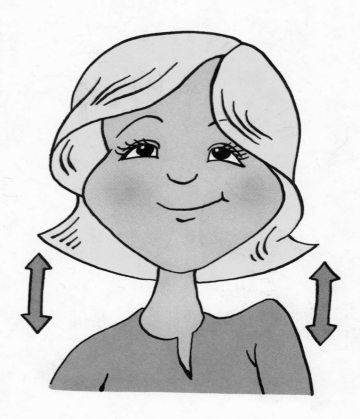

4. Sit with head hanging forward, chin pressed against the chest. Keep the chin in position and as if bending the head backward as far as it will go, look toward the ceiling. Return. Repeat the exercise fifteen times.

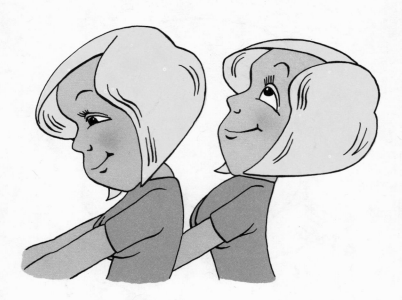

EXERCISE PROGRAM

D

In front of the TV

1. Sit with feet parallel, pointing straight ahead. Lift the left leg up against the chest and clasp the lower leg with both hands. Pull! Return to original position. Repeat the same movement with the right leg. Lift up both knees and clasp both hands around the lower legs. Pull! Return to original position. Raise your body from the seat until the buttocks just clear the seat cushion, at the same time rolling the feet up onto the toes. Return to original position. Relax. Repeat the exercise five times.

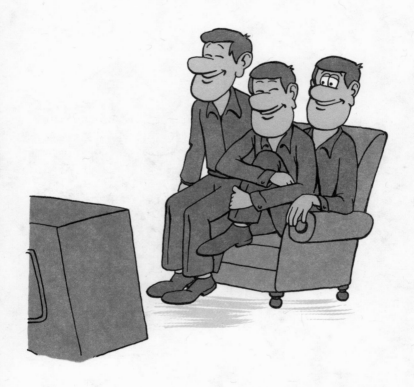

2. Sit relaxed. Alternate tensing and relaxing of lower back muscles. Concentrate on tensing only the lower back muscles and keeping all other muscles relaxed. Repeat the exercise fifteen times.

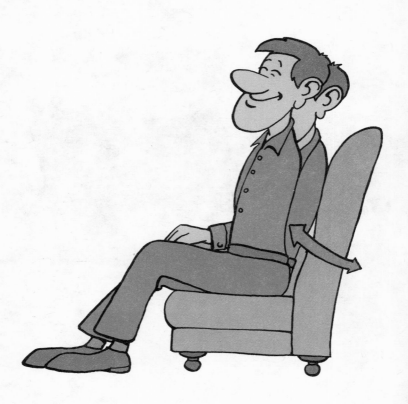

3. Sit with shoulders dropped. Pull the shoulder blades firmly together behind the back with shoulders still dropped. Draw the elbows backward. Move the shoulders forward, folding arms over each other. Relax. Repeat the exercise eight times.

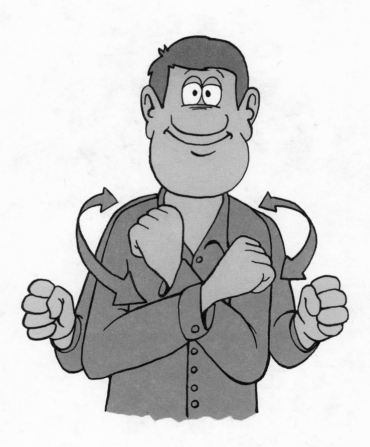

4. Sit with arms crossed—the right hand on the left shoulder, the left hand on the right shoulder. Bend the head to the left until the left ear touches the right hand. Return to original position. Now bend the head to the right so that the right ear touches the left hand. Return. Repeat the exercise eight times.

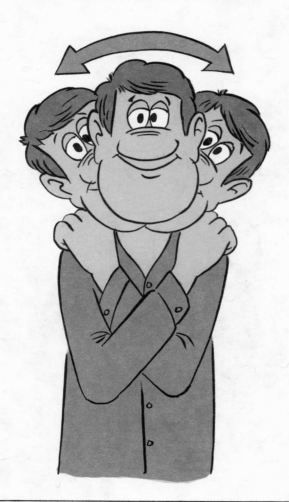

EXERCISE PROGRAM

E

On the Train or Bus

1. Sit with the elbows on the knees and the whole weight of the body pressing down on the knees. Move your feet to the right with a zigzag motion, lifting first the heels and then the toes. Make four zigzag steps. Then make four of the same steps to the left. Repeat the exercise eight times.

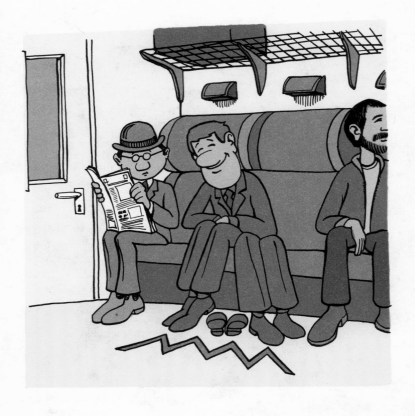

2. Sit relaxed. Pull the stomach muscles in as far as you can. Keep them drawn in, tensed for seven seconds. Relax for seven seconds. Repeat the exercise eight times.

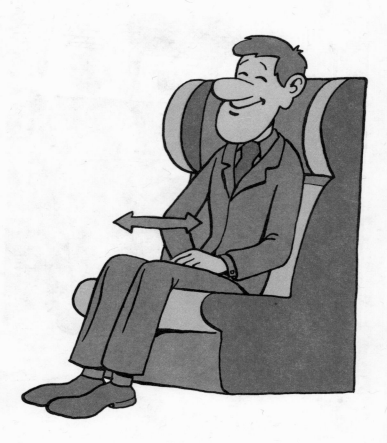

3. Sit with shoulders dropped. Move the right shoulder forward, then the left shoulder forward, stretching each as you do so. Return. Relax. Clasp the hands and move the arms upward, then backward as the palms are turned upward, giving a slight pull backward. Repeat the exercise eight times.

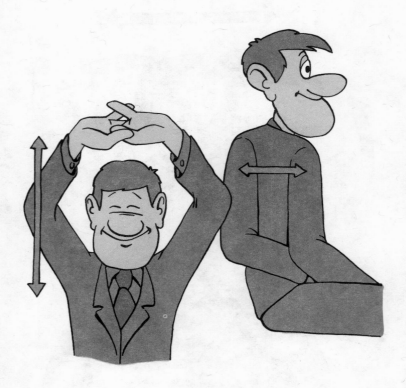

4. Sit with the head facing front. Turn the head horizontally all the way to the left. Bend the head all the way forward, as if nodding. Raise the head again. Turn the head forward again. Do the same exercise, turning the head toward the right. Repeat both left and right exercises eight times.

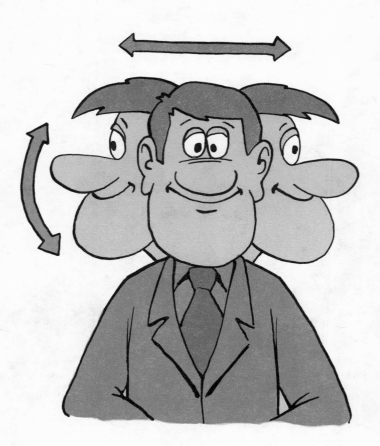

EXERCISE PROGRAM
F
In the Office or at School

1. Sit with toes on the floor, heels high in the air, toes tucked well in toward the chair. Stretch out the left knee as far as possible while pushing the heel forward and drawing the toes as far toward you as possible. Return to original position. Relax. Repeat the same movement with the right leg. Repeat the same movement with both legs together. Do left, right, and both leg exercises four times.

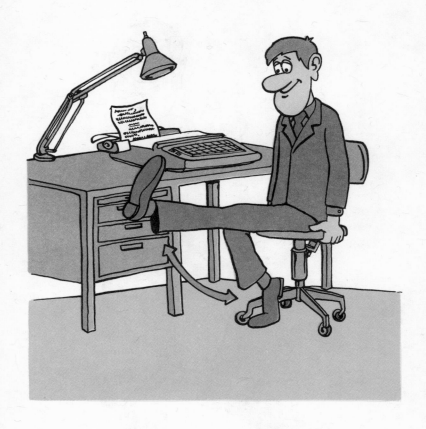

2. Sit with arms folded and feet together. Move the right foot forward one step. At the same time, pivot your body to the right, adding an extra stretch at the end. Change feet, and at the same time pivot your body to the left, again with an extra stretch. Repeat the exercise eight times.

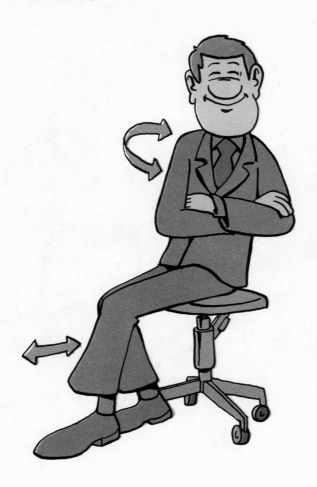

3. Sit with shoulders dropped. Grasp the left shoulder with the right hand and the right shoulder with the left hand. Return. Relax. Place both hands behind the neck. Return. Relax. Try to reach the elbow of the opposite arm behind the back—first with the left hand, then with the right. Return. Relax. Repeat the exercise eight times.

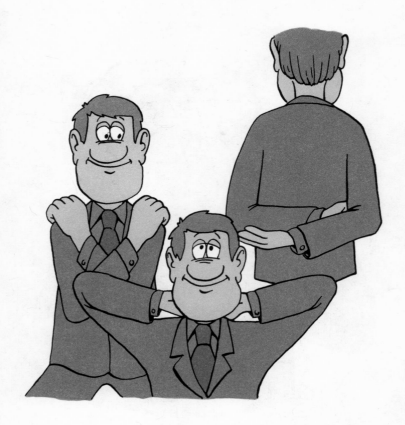

4. Sit with right hand against the head above the right ear. Bend the head straight to the right, offering a slight resistance with the hand. Return. Repeat the same movement with the left hand above the left ear. Repeat the exercise eight times.

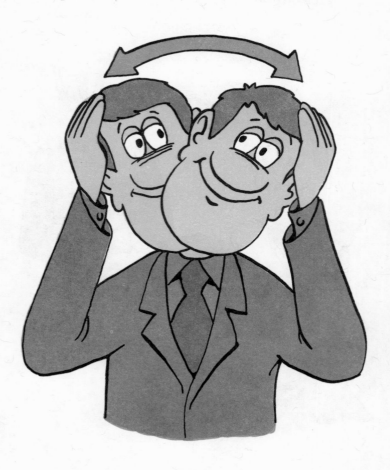

EXERCISE PROGRAM

G

In the Waiting Room

1. Sit with the toes pointed on the floor and the heels high. Point knees to the right and drop them all the way down on the heel. Then, on toes again, point knees to the left and drop them down. Alternate this movement twice. Stretch both legs out as far as possible, pulling the toes as far forward toward your body as they will go. Return. Repeat the forward stretch. Repeat the whole exercise four times.

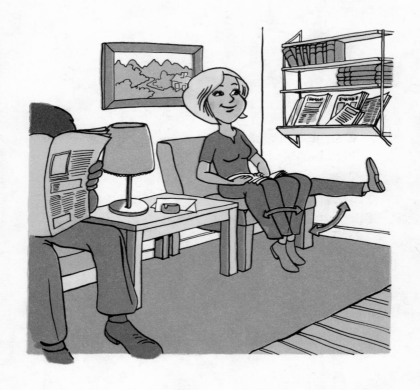

2. Sit with your lower legs crossed tightly below the knee. Make sideways bends from the waist alternately to the left and to the right. Give a gentle extra push at the end of each bend. Repeat the exercise eight times.

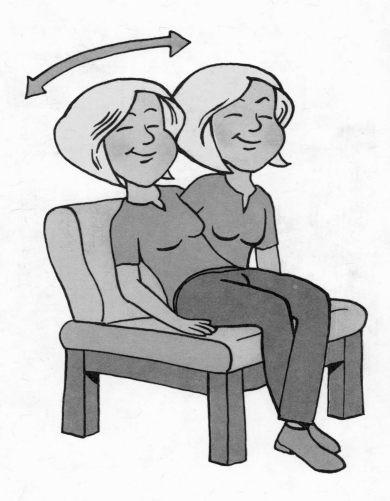

3. Sit with shoulders dropped. Stretch one arm upward, the other arm outward. Push each as far as you can. Return to starting position. Relax. Repeat the exercise, raising your arms in different directions, alternating the upwards arm. Repeat the whole exercise eight times.

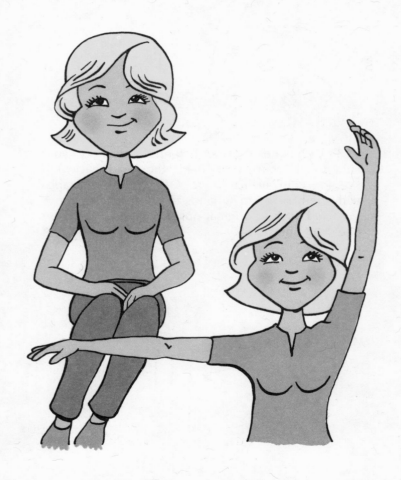

4. Sit with hands together behind the neck. Let your chin touch your chest. Bend the head backward keeping chin against chest. Offer slight resistance with the hands. Move hands to the forehead. Move the head back to original position. Repeat the exercise eight times.

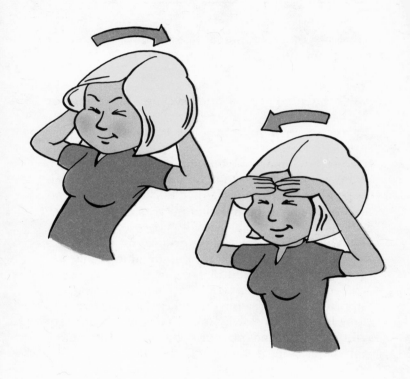

ᴖere are some additional tips on how to keep fit while you are using the *Exercises in the Chair* program:

1. Exercise your whole body two or three times a week by running, walking, cycling, swimming, or similar activity.

2. Keep your limbs and joints in trim with regular exercise sessions or ballet—rhythmic movements using the full range of your joints.

3. At work and play exercise your muscles as often as possible, trying to use a rhythmic pattern of movements in which the muscles are tensed and relaxed alternately for equal periods.

4. Whenever you feel tense or anxious, try the following exercise: Sit fully relaxed. Breathe evenly and gently, using so-called diaphragm breathing, which comes from deep down. This involves filling the stomach when breathing in, which is an active motion. Breathe out slowly; this is a passive motion. Let all the air out, and let your body sink into complete relaxation. Repeat the exercise five times.

I wish you happy—and healthy—sitting!

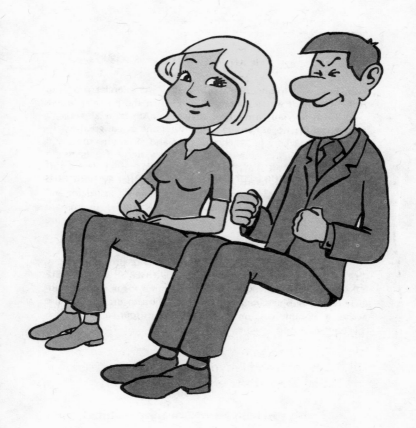

ABOUT THE AUTHORS

Even before his pioneering work on the SAS exercise program, *Folke Mossfeldt* was a leading researcher in the physical fitness field. He is not only a medical adviser to SAS: he is also a staff member of the Royal Karolinska Institute, one of the great teaching hospitals, where he teaches doctors and physiotherapists and consults on specific exercises for a wide variety of patients. In 1959, he pioneered special exercises for patients who have suffered strokes and heart attacks, a therapy that is now used around the world. Mr. Mossfeldt has also been ski instructor and physical trainer for King Carl Gustaf and his family. His exercise programs on Swedish TV have made him a popular figure throughout that country.

Mary Susan Miller is the co-author of two previous books, STRAIGHT TALK TO PARENTS and A TEACHER'S ROUNDTABLE ON SEX EDUCATION. Ms. Miller has written for numerous publications on subjects ranging from education to drama. She also writes a monthly column for *Ladies' Home Journal* called "Between Parent And Teacher."